▲ Describe blood components and blood products

▲ Explain blood group compatibility and the significance of the ABO and Rh blood group system

▲ Demonstrate the safe administration of blood

▲ Identify blood transfusion complications, reactions, and steps for management of reactions

▲ Apply the 8 Rights of Blood Administration

Review the **A L E R T** boxes throughout the handbook to understand why it is important not to deviate from recommended practices.

The ![HOSPITAL] icon is used to remind you to consult your hospital policy for information specific to your facility as practice may vary from hospital to hospital.

Throughout this handbook, TML refers to the Transfusion Medicine Laboratory in your hospital, sometimes referred to as the Blood Bank or Transfusion Service.

Definitions

▲ The term **Blood Component** in this handbook refers to a therapeutic component of blood intended for transfusion (e.g., red blood cells, platelets, plasma) that can be prepared using the equipment and techniques available in a blood centre

▲ The term **Blood Product** in this handbook refers to any therapeutic product, derived from human blood or plasma, and produced by a manufacturing process that pools multiple units (e.g., albumin, immunoglobulin and coagulation products)

D1253159

3

Who regulates?

Health Canada regulates blood collection, testing, processing, and distribution.

Who collects?

Canadian Blood Services (CBS) collects, tests donor blood and distributes blood components and products in all provinces and territories, except Quebec (Héma-Québec).

National Standards

- ▲ National standards for blood and blood components are developed by the Canadian Standards Association (CSA)
- ▲ The Canadian Society for Transfusion Medicine (CSTM) also publishes standards for hospital transfusion services

CONTENTS

ABO blood group system

Blood groups are genetically determined. In the ABO system, the A and B antigens are either present or absent on the surface of an individual's red blood cells (RBCs). Starting at about four months of age, ABO antibodies have been naturally acquired to the antigens absent from a person's red blood cells. These antibodies are found in the individual's plasma.

For example, group A people will have the A antigen on their red blood cell (RBC) surface and will produce anti-B antibody because they lack the B antigen. The anti-B is found in their plasma.

Group	ABO antigen on red blood cell	Frequency	ABO antibody in plasma
A	A	40%	anti-B
B	B	11%	anti-A
AB	A and B	4%	None
O	None	45%	anti-A and anti-B

Compatibility

The patient's ABO group is the most important blood group system used to determine compatibility for a blood transfusion. Patients must receive blood components that are ABO compatible but not necessarily identical to their own blood group.

See *Appendix 3 – **Compatibility chart***.

Compatibility of a blood component is determined by the antigens and antibodies present in the recipient and the donor component.

A patient's antibodies will hemolyse transfused RBCs that have the corresponding antigen on their surface. For example:

▲ A patient who is group O (having anti-A and anti-B antibodies) will hemolyse the blood being transfused if they are transfused with group A or group B RBCs

Donor antibodies in plasma components (and occasionally IVIG) can hemolyse a patient's RBCs if they have the corresponding antigen.

▲ Plasma from a group B donor (containing anti-A antibodies) can hemolyse a group A patient's RBCs

In both cases the resulting potentially fatal reaction is a Hemolytic Transfusion Reaction.

Rh blood group system

The Rh system, also known as the Rhesus system, is the second most important of the blood group systems. The Rh antigen, commonly, referred to as the "D" antigen is either present [Rh(D) positive] or lacking [Rh(D) negative] on the surface of the red blood cell.

Rh negative patients can develop an antibody to Rh(D) if they are exposed to Rh positive red blood cells. This sensitization can occur through transfusion of Rh positive RBCs or platelets (which may contain small amounts of red blood cells) and during pregnancy. Pregnant Rh negative females may develop the Rh(D) antibody by exposure to small amounts of blood from an Rh(D) positive fetus during pregnancy and at delivery.

▲ Rh Immune Globulin (RhIG) is given during pregnancy and after delivery to prevent development of Rh(D) antibodies

Once present, Rh(D) antibodies in the mother will cross the placenta and hemolyse the red blood cells of any future Rh positive fetus. This results in anemia, jaundice, brain damage, or even death of the fetus and is known as Hemolytic Disease of the Fetus and Newborn (HDFN).

Rh negative females of child-bearing potential (less than 45 years of age) should not be exposed to Rh positive RBCs in order to prevent the development of the Rh(D) antibody.

Plasma and cryoprecipitate units do not contain any RBCs and so cannot expose the patient to the Rh(D) antigen. The Rh group of plasma and cryoprecipitate is irrelevant for transfusion.

See *Appendix 3* – **Compatibility chart**.

Notes

Urgent transfusions:
Prior to blood group confirmation

Historically

Patients whose blood group was unknown, and who required an urgent transfusion, would be provided with Group O Rh negative RBCs until the patient's blood group was determined.

In recent years

▲ Demand for group O Rh negative RBCs exceeds the supply

▲ There is a chronic shortage of O Rh negative RBCs

In situations where the blood group is unknown:

▲ The TML will usually issue O Rh negative RBCs for females of child bearing potential (less than 45 years of age) until the patient's blood group is confirmed

▲ All males and women past child bearing potential can receive O Rh positive RBCs until the patient's blood group is confirmed

This practice carries minimal risk to the patient.

Informed consent

Prior to transfusing a patient, consent should be obtained by the health care professional prescribing the treatment. Consent must be documented on the patient's chart prior to transfusion.

The transfusion consent usually remains in effect for the entire admission or course of treatment. Consent should be obtained before the patient's blood specimen is collected.

Continued on the next page...

Informed consent (cont'd)

Transfusion can be given without consent only if the following conditions exist (refer to hospital policy and procedure for transfusion without consent):

- ▲ Urgent transfusion needed to preserve life or continuing health **AND**

- ▲ Patient unable to consent and substitute decision maker is not available **AND**

- ▲ No evidence of prior wishes refusing transfusion for personal or religious reasons

Guidelines for the person obtaining consent from patient or substitute decision maker:

- ▲ Provide information about the blood component/product, including the benefits of the transfusion, and reason the transfusion is required

- ▲ Describe the risks of the transfusion, including non-infectious and infectious risks. This discussion should include the risks of not receiving a transfusion

- ▲ Discuss alternatives that are appropriate for the patient's medical condition

- ▲ When possible, consent for transfusion should be discussed early enough to allow for blood alternatives to be considered

- ▲ Provide the patient with the opportunity to ask questions. Patient information pamphlets can be used but should not replace the need for a discussion with a health care professional obtaining consent

- ▲ Document that consent was obtained according to your institutional policy AND clearly document the reason for transfusion in the patient's chart

- ▲ In Ontario, there is no legal age of consent. Pediatric patients may give informed consent if they have the capacity to understand the information about the treatment and the risks of not having the treatment. A parent or legal guardian may give consent for minors deemed not to have the capacity. It is important to note that the age at which informed consent can be given may vary from province to province. Refer to provincial legislation

Transfusion orders

Transfusions must be ordered by a physician or authorized practitioner.

All orders must include:

▲ Patient's first and last name and at least one unique identifier

▲ Blood component or product type

▲ Number of units or amount

▲ Rate of infusion

▲ Special requirements if any (e.g., irradiated)

▲ Premedication or diuretic, if required

It has been shown that non-urgent transfusions should occur during daytime hours for increased patient safety.

Example of a physician's transfusion order:

> John Doe
> Hospital Number 2345678
>
> March 10, 2015 @ 2130
>
> In AM, transfuse one unit irradiated red blood cells over 3 hours.
> Furosemide 20 mg IV pre-transfusion.
> Repeat CBC and contact physician to assess for further transfusion needs.
>
> Dr. J. Stevens

Notes

Requesting the blood component/product

Prior to requesting the blood component/product:

▲ Review the most recent laboratory values. The following blood tests may be used to monitor the need for and/or effectiveness of transfusion:

Blood Component/Product	Laboratory Blood Test
Red blood cell (RBC)	Hemoglobin
Platelet	Platelet count
Frozen Plasma (FP) and Prothrombin Complex Concentrate (PCC)	International Normalized Ratio (INR)
Cryoprecipitate	Fibrinogen

▲ Assess the patient's symptoms

▲ Know the indications and appropriate dosage to verify that the transfusion is appropriate

- See *Appendix 1* – **Blood components table** and *Appendix 2* – **Blood products table**

When requesting blood from the TML, the following items are required:

▲ Patient's first and last name along with one additional unique identifier

▲ Patient's location

▲ Diagnosis/special blood component preparation instructions (such as irradiation)

▲ Blood component/product required

▲ Amount/dose

▲ Time required

▲ Prescriber's name

Additional information may be required:

▲ History of recent blood exposure – usually through transfusion or pregnancy

▲ Indication or reason for transfusion

▲ Patient's weight (for pediatric patients and orders for IVIG)

▲ If ordering by electronic order entry, ensure the order is entered for the correct patient and the correct blood component/product. If processing is manual, ensure legible and appropriate paperwork is taken or sent to the TML. This ensures the correct component/product is retrieved for the correct patient and prevents any delays in preparation

Notes

_____

_____

_____

_____

_____

_____

_____

_____

Pre-transfusion samples

Determine if a pre-transfusion sample is required. The expiry or outdate of a sample will vary depending on the patient's recent blood exposure, pregnancy history, and previous antibody screen results. The age of very young pediatric patients may also be a factor.

Pre-transfusion samples (commonly referred to as a Group and Screen or Type and Screen) are used to:

▲ Determine ABO and Rh blood groups (i.e., group/type)

▲ Detect and identify antibodies acquired from previous blood exposure or pregnancy (i.e., screen)

▲ Crossmatch suitable units of blood when a transfusion is ordered

Patient Identification:

1. Check the patient's arm band or identification to make sure it is the correct patient, EVEN when the patient is familiar to you. Assuming you know the patient can greatly increase the risk of wrong patient identification.

2. When possible, include the patient/parent in the identification process by asking specific questions. It is not recommended to use questions that only require only a Yes or No answer (e.g., "Are you John Smith?"). Use questions such as:

   • "How do you spell your name?"
   • "What is your date of birth?"

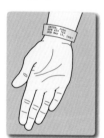

If any discrepancies are discovered, they must be resolved prior to collecting a pre-transfusion sample.

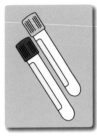

4 steps for labeling samples:

1. Take sample labels with you to your patient's bedside

2. Verify that the labels match the patient's armband/identification and any accompanying paperwork

3. After collecting the blood sample(s), label the tubes <u>before</u> leaving the patient's bedside

   • **Never label samples away from the patient, which greatly increases the risk of mislabeling**

4. Document that you drew the blood sample. Never sign for a sample collected by your colleague

Accurate patient identification is critical.

▲ Misidentified patients can result in incompatible blood being transfused to the patient

Accurate labeling of a pre-transfusion sample is critical.

▲ Mislabeled samples can result in a patient receiving incompatible blood

A L E R T

Accurate patient identification is as critical with sample draws as it is when administering blood components/products.

Preparing the patient

Explain the purpose and monitoring for the transfusion.
Ensure that the patient's questions are addressed.

Determine if your patient has had any problems or reactions
with previous transfusions. If so, orders from a physician for
premedication may be required:

▲ IV route – Administer immediately pre-transfusion

▲ po route – Administer 30 minutes pre-transfusion

Indication	Premedication
Repeated allergic reactions	Antihistamine and/or steroid
Repeated febrile reactions	Antipyretic

*Meperidine - Demerol® is not
indicated as a premedication*

IV access

Determine the correct IV access required:

Blood Component/Product	IV Access
Red blood cells – rapid transfusions in adults	16-18G (Gauge)
Red blood cells – routine transfusions in adults	20-22G
Other blood components/products	Any size is adequate
Pediatrics	22-25G
All components and products – adults and pediatrics	Central venous access devices (CVAD)

Transfusing rapidly and under pressure through too small an IV access can cause hemolysis of RBCs.

Ensure that the IV access is dedicated to the transfusion.

Blood components/products must not come in contact with medications or incompatible solutions.

When transfusing through a CVAD with multiple lumens, medications/solutions can be infused through other lumens without damaging the blood component/product.

IV pumps, blood warmers, and rapid infusers must be suitable for transfusion and not damage the blood component/product. Do not use devices that have not been approved for use with blood components/products.

Blood tubing

The following blood components must be transfused through blood tubing containing a 170-260 micron filter to capture any fibrin debris:

▲ RBC, platelets, plasma, cryosupernatant plasma and cryoprecipitate

Flush blood tubing with normal saline (0.9% NaCl), completely wetting filter. For small pediatric patients, the blood tubing may be primed with the blood component instead of saline due to concerns for volume overload.

Blood tubing must be changed at least every 2-4 units and within the number of hours specified by your hospital policy.

In cases of massive transfusion, an add-on filter can be used to minimize the frequency of tubing changes.

Note that:

Platelets are best transfused through blood tubing not previously used for RBC. Platelets will adhere to fibrin captured in the filter.

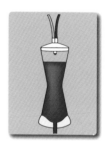

Blood products (such as IVIG and albumin) do not require blood tubing or a blood filter. IV tubing that can be vented is required for IV infusions directly from glass bottles.

Some IVIG brands may not be compatible with normal saline. Refer to package insert or specific hospital guidelines.

Notes

Picking up blood

BEFORE picking up blood, ensure that the patient is ready:

▲ Connect the primed IV tubing to the patient's IV site to ensure patency

▲ Verify that consent for transfusion has been obtained and that there is a written order for the transfusion

▲ Administer any premedication that may be ordered – generally only recommended for patients who have previously experienced repeated transfusion reactions

Arrange for pickup or delivery from the TML using appropriate documentation to ensure the correct unit is retrieved for the correct patient.

If the transfusion cannot be started immediately contact the TML or refer to hospital policy.

<u>Never</u> store blood in unapproved fridges such as medication or ward fridges.

Properly identify patient:

▲ All patients being transfused must be wearing an ID armband or be identified using an alternate form of identification approved by your hospital

ALERT

Blood must be started soon after it is received and completed within 4 hours of removal from proper storage to decrease the risk of bacterial contamination.

ALERT

Blood components/products must only be stored in areas (equipment) where temperatures are monitored specifically for blood components/products.

Notes

_____

_____

_____

_____

_____

_____

_____

_____

Checking blood

▲ Visually check the blood unit for clots, unusual colour and any leaks

▲ Check the expiration date on the Canadian Blood Services (CBS) label

  • See *Appendix 4* – **Canadian Blood Services label**

▲ Check the patient's ABO and Rh (when available). Ensure the donor's blood group is compatible for the patient

  • See *Appendix 3* – **Compatibility chart**

▲ Check the transfusion order for component/product type and volume required and verify that consent was obtained

ALWAYS check blood at the patient's bedside.

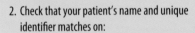

Steps for checking blood:

1. Check your patient's armband to make sure it is correct. When possible, include your patient or parents (if pediatric) in the identification process by asking specific questions:

  • "How do you spell your name?"
  • "What is your date of birth?"

2. Check that your patient's name and unique identifier matches on:

  • ID armband
  • TML label/tag attached to blood

3. Check that the blood unit number and donor blood group matches on:

  • CBS label
  • TML label/tag attached to blood

If you find any discrepancies, do not proceed. Contact the TML immediately.

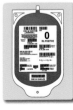

Continued on the next page...

Checking blood (cont'd)

To avoid errors, most hospitals have two qualified individuals complete the pre-transfusion check.

Blood must be started soon after being received and immediately after being checked.

The TML label/tag must remain attached to the blood unit throughout the transfusion.

The chart copy of the TML label or tag should be placed in the patient's chart, according to your hospital policy.

A L E R T

Checking blood immediately prior to the transfusion is the last opportunity to catch any errors.

Notes

_____

_____

_____

_____

_____

_____

_____

_____

_____

Starting blood

Before starting blood:

Record baseline vital signs and assessment before starting each unit:

- ▲ Temperature
- ▲ Blood pressure
- ▲ Pulse
- ▲ Respiration
- ▲ Oxygen saturation if available
- ▲ Auscultation for patients at risk for overload (elderly, pediatric, cardiovascular disease)

Steps for spiking blood:

1. Separate the port cover until port is exposed
2. Port covers that are not removable must be held away from the port to prevent contamination
3. Hold the blood bag in one hand and exposed blood tubing spike in the other. Do not hang from the IV pole
4. Insert blood tubing spike into port while pushing gently and turning clock-wise with ¼ turns. Do not over-spike. Spiking properly will ensure easy removal of the blood bag if required
5. To remove bag, pull gently while turning the spike counter-clockwise

Continued on the next page…

Starting blood (cont'd)

Steps for spiking blood products supplied in glass bottles (IVIG, albumin):

1. Remove the seal to expose port and swab with alcohol
2. Close roller clamp on IV tubing
3. Place bottle on a flat surface and spike at a 90° angle through the center circle of the stopper
4. Invert and hang bottle on IV pole
5. Squeeze drip chamber to ½ full
6. Open vent on drip chamber – this allows air to enter the bottle
7. Open roller clamp and prime remainder of tubing
8. Close vent prior to spiking each subsequent bottle, then hang bottle and open vent

After starting blood:

1. For the first 15 minutes:
   - Start initially with a slow rate unless transfusion is extremely urgent
   - Monitor your patient closely
2. After the first 15 minutes:
   - Reassess your patient and repeat vital signs
   - Increase flow to prescribed rate if no reaction observed

HOSPITAL **Notes**

Monitoring

Monitor, Monitor, Monitor!

Monitor the patient closely and document vital signs:

▲ Prior to the transfusion – within previous 30 minutes

▲ After the first 15 minutes of the blood unit

▲ At prescribed intervals, according to your hospital policy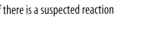

▲ At the end of the unit

▲ If there is a suspected reaction

Repeat with each subsequent unit.

Repeat vital signs more often for patients:

▲ At greater risk for circulatory overload (elderly, pediatric, cardiovascular disease)

▲ Who have experienced previous reactions

▲ Who are already unstable

When possible, instruct your patient to notify you if they experience:

▲ Hives or itching

▲ Feeling feverish or chills

▲ Difficulty breathing

▲ Back pain or pain at the infusion site

▲ Any feeling different from usual

Continued on the next page...

Monitoring (cont'd)

Massive Transfusions

A massive transfusion is defined as more than 10 units of RBCs, or, transfusing more than one blood volume in a 24-hour period.

Recommendations for the management of patients during massive transfusion/bleeding include:

▲ Monitor core temperature

▲ Prompt use of measures to prevent hypothermia, including use of a blood warmer for all IV fluids and RBC and plasma transfusions

▲ Monitor for dilutional coagulopathy

▲ While patient is actively bleeding, transfuse to keep:

• Hemoglobin greater than 70g/L

• Platelet count greater than 50 X 10^9/L (if head injury - greater than 100 X 10^9/L)

• INR less than 1.5-2.0

• Fibrinogen greater than 2.0g/L

▲ Consider the use of tranexamic acid

▲ Monitor for hypocalcemia, acidosis and hyperkalemia

A L E R T

For children over 4 months old, the estimated blood volume is 70 ml/kg. The estimated blood volume for a neonate is 80-100 ml/kg.

Completing a transfusion

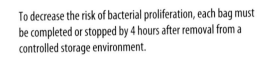

Guidelines for completing a transfusion:

1. Complete transfusion within 4 hours of removal from controlled storage

2. If desired, flush the blood tubing with normal saline

3. Disconnect blood tubing when transfusion is completed

4. Check end of transfusion vital signs

5. Repeat vital signs periodically post transfusion according to your hospital policy

To decrease the risk of bacterial proliferation, each bag must be completed or stopped by 4 hours after removal from a controlled storage environment.

Used blood tubing can breed bacteria. Do not leave it attached to the patient.

Dispose of used blood tubing and blood bags in a biohazard container unless your hospital policy requires you to return the blood bags to the TML.

Continue to assess the patient for symptoms of reactions that might occur up to 6 hours post transfusion.

Notes

Out-patients or their care givers should be provided with an information sheet detailing:

▲ Signs and symptoms of transfusion reactions

▲ Information on what to do when experiencing a reaction and when to seek medical attention

▲ Contact information for reporting reactions

Documentation

Document each blood transfusion by placing the blood transfusion record (or a copy) in the patient's chart.

The record should include:

▲ Date

▲ Start and finish times

▲ Type of component/product transfused

▲ Blood unit number or lot number

▲ Name of persons starting and checking blood

Additional information should be documented in the patient's chart:

▲ Vital signs and patient assessments

▲ Volume transfused

▲ Follow-up testing done:
  • CBC after RBC or platelet transfusion, if required
  • INR, PT/PTT after plasma
  • Fibrinogen level after cryoprecipitate

▲ Patient teaching

▲ Any reactions and treatment provided

Some hospitals require the return of a transfusion form to the TML.

Notes

Recognizing reactions

Acute reactions usually occur during or up to 6 hours following the end of a transfusion and may present with:

- ▲ Fever
- ▲ Shaking chills or rigors with or without fever
- ▲ Hives or rash, itchiness, swelling
- ▲ Dyspnea, shortness of breath or wheezing
- ▲ Hypotension or hypertension
- ▲ Red urine, diffuse bleeding or oozing
- ▲ Lumbar pain, anxiety, pain at the IV site
- ▲ Nausea and vomiting
- ▲ Headache
- ▲ Irritability in pediatric population

Initially it can be challenging to distinguish a minor reaction from a serious reaction based solely on the presenting signs and symptoms.

Any unexpected or suspicious symptom should be reported to the TML for investigation of a possible transfusion reaction.

Chest X-ray of a patient before and during an episode of transfusion-related acute lung injury (TRALI)

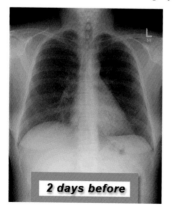

2 days before

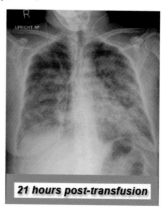

21 hours post-transfusion

Acute transfusion reactions

Acute transfusion reactions may present with similar signs and symptoms.

Signs and Symptoms	Possible Transfusion Reaction
Fever, chills or rigors	▲ Bacterial contamination ▲ Acute hemolytic transfusion reaction ▲ Transfusion-related acute lung injury (TRALI) ▲ Febrile non-hemolytic transfusion reaction
Urticaria and other allergic symptoms	▲ Anaphylaxis ▲ Minor allergic reaction
Dyspnea	▲ TRALI ▲ Transfusion-associated circulatory overload (TACO) ▲ Anaphylaxis ▲ Bacterial contamination ▲ Acute hemolytic transfusion reaction
Hypertension	▲ TACO
Hypotension	▲ Bradykinin mediated hypotension ▲ Bacterial contamination ▲ Acute hemolytic transfusion reaction ▲ TRALI ▲ Anaphylaxis
Hemolysis, red urine (hemoglobinuria)	▲ Acute hemolytic transfusion reaction
Pain	▲ Acute hemolytic transfusion reaction • IV site • Lumbar ▲ TACO • Chest
Nausea and vomiting	▲ Acute hemolytic transfusion reaction ▲ Anaphylaxis ▲ Febrile non hemolytic transfusion reaction

See Appendix 5 – **Acute reactions - risk and description table** *for risk of event and description.*

Acute reaction management

Suspected reaction management:

1. Stop the transfusion immediately!

2. Maintain IV access for treatment if necessary but do not flush the blood tubing

3. Check vital signs

4. Verify that patient ID matches the TML tag/label

5. Verify that the blood unit number matches the TML tag/label

6. Notify the physician but remain with the patient

7. Notify the TML of the reaction as per hospital policy

8. Treat patient's symptoms as ordered by the physician

If the patient experiences minor allergic or minor febrile symptoms only, restarting the transfusion may be possible. Refer to your hospital policy for guidelines.

General guidelines for continuing a transfusion:

▲ Consult physician

▲ Medicate patient as ordered

▲ Proceed cautiously with more frequent patient assessments

▲ Remember 4 hour limit

▲ Report to TML if required but further investigation is not necessary

Reaction investigation

To investigate a reaction, the following may be required by the TML:

1. Blood bag with attached blood tubing for:
   - Possible culture
   - Hemolysis check
   - Clerical check

2. Previously infused blood bags if available

3. Transfusion reaction reporting document with:
   - Symptoms
   - Pre and post vital signs
   - Time of onset
   - Blood unit number or lot number

4. Post transfusion blood sample with required paperwork for:
   - Repeat group/type and screen, and repeat crossmatch for comparison with pre transfusion testing results
   - Direct antiglobulin test (DAT)
   - Hemolysis check

Continued on the next page…

Notes

_____

_____

_____

_____

_____

_____

_____

_____

Reaction investigation (cont'd)

Depending on patient signs and symptoms, additional testing may be required:

- ▲ Next voided urine for hemoglobin testing:
  - • Monitor urine output if hemolysis suspected
- ▲ Chest x-ray if patient has new respiratory symptoms
- ▲ Blood cultures from the patient:
  - • Drawn from a different vein
  - • Antibiotics should be started immediately if bacterial sepsis suspected
  - • Report immediately to the TML as the blood supplier/manufacturer must be alerted
- ▲ Other blood samples may be required to investigate:
  - • Anaphylactic reactions
  - • TRALI
  - • Acute hemolytic transfusion reaction

The TML must report serious reactions to blood components/products to the manufacturer or the Canada Vigilance Program. Other components/products may be implicated and need to be recalled.

The TML may also report reactions to Ontario Transfusion Transmitted Injuries Surveillance System (TTISS-ON), which collects transfusion reaction data in order to monitor and improve transfusion safety for all patients.

See Appendix 6 – **Transfusion reaction chart** *for recommended investigations, treatment and actions.*

8 Rights of Transfusion

1. Right patient

▲ Pay meticulous attention to patient identification when collecting/labeling pre-transfusion samples

▲ Match the patient's name and unique identifier on the blood component/product with the order in the chart

▲ At the bedside, confirm that the patient's name and unique identifier on the blood component/product match the name and unique identifier on their armband (or other form of positive ID)

▲ Whenever possible, include the patient during the identification process

2. Right blood component/product

▲ Confirm that blood component/product is appropriate for the indication for transfusion

▲ Ensure the blood component/product label matches the orders (e.g., the orders are for irradiated RBC)

▲ Visually inspect and ensure blood component/product is not damaged

▲ Check expiry date/time

3. Right reason

▲ Confirm the diagnosis and/or indication for transfusion

▲ Review latest lab values and patient symptoms to ensure the transfusion is indicated and within hospital guidelines

4. Right dose

▲ Verify that the dose is appropriate for the patient's condition

▲ Verify that the dose is appropriate for the patient's weight (e.g., pediatric patients or orders for IVIG)

▲ Consider if patient is at high risk for circulatory overload (e.g., pediatric, elderly, compromised cardiac function)

Continued on the next page...

8 Rights of Transfusion (cont'd)

5. Right time

- ▲ Ensure that the component/product will be initiated as soon as it is received from the TML
- ▲ Ensure that the transfusion will be completed within four hours from the time of issue
- ▲ Begin transfusion slowly for first 15 minutes
- ▲ Ensure rate of transfusion is appropriate for patient's status (e.g., pediatric, elderly, compromised cardiac function)

6. Right site

- ▲ Ensure there is a patent IV prior to retrieving blood so that the blood component/product can be started as soon as received
- ▲ Dedicated access is required for transfusion
- ▲ Medications and IV solutions other than normal saline can cause hemolysis or clotting of the transfused blood
- ▲ Change blood tubing according to hospital policy to decrease potential for growth of any bacteria and discard when complete

7. Right documentation

- ▲ Ensure physician's order is documented
- ▲ Verify consent for transfusion has been obtained and documented
- ▲ Document vital signs at a minimum before starting transfusion, 15 minutes after the start, and upon completion (and at prescribed intervals according to your hospital policy)
- ▲ Document start and stop times
- ▲ Document any changes in patient's condition or signs/symptoms of transfusion reaction

8. Right response

- ▲ Recognize and treat adverse reactions appropriately
- ▲ Report reactions to the TML to ensure proper investigation and notification of the blood supplier/manufacturer
- ▲ Review post transfusion bloodwork if required to assess effectiveness of the transfusion and re-assess patient's symptoms

Policies and procedures at different facilities may vary.

Sources for more information...

- ▲ Bloody Easy Blood Administration eLearning – www.transfusionontario.org
- ▲ Bloody Easy for Physicians eLearning – www.transfusionontario.org
- ▲ Bloody Easy 3 Handbook www.transfusionontario.org
- ▲ Blood Transfusion – Information For Patients www.transfusionontario.org
- ▲ Canadian Society for Transfusion Medicine – Choosing Wisely Canada http://www.transfusion.ca/en/choosing_wisely

Appendix 1: Blood components table

Blood Components	Major Uses	Storage & Expiration	Administration
Red Blood Cells (RBC)	Bleeding or anemic non-bleeding patients with signs and symptoms of impaired tissue oxygen delivery. ▲ Tachycardia ▲ Shortness of breath ▲ Dizziness	2-6° C in approved fridge only **Up to 42 days**	▲ Blood tubing required ▲ Initiate transfusion slowly for first 15 minutes unless massive blood loss ▲ Transfuse over no more than 4 hours ▲ Typically over 1 ½ - 2 hours with slower rates for patients at risk for circulatory overload
Plasma	▲ Liver disease coagulopathy ▲ Massive transfusion ▲ Plasma exchange procedures for certain diseases (e.g., Thrombotic Thrombocytopenic Purpura/Hemolytic Uremic Syndrome)	Frozen **1 year** Once thawed expires after 5 days stored at 1-6° C	▲ Blood tubing required ▲ Initiate transfusion slowly for first 15 minutes unless massive blood loss ▲ Transfuse over no more than 4 hours ▲ Typically over 30 minutes - 2 hours

Blood Components	Major Uses	Storage & Expiration	Administration
Platelets	Control or prevent bleeding in patients with: ▲ Low platelet counts (Thrombocytopenia) ▲ Congenital platelet dysfunction ▲ Platelets not functioning due to the effects of medications (ASA, Clopidogrel - Plavix®) ▲ Platelet dysfunction following cardiopulmonary bypass	20-24° C on an agitator to prevent clumping 5 days	▲ Blood tubing required ▲ New blood tubing recommended ▲ Initiate transfusion slowly for first 15 minutes unless massive blood loss ▲ Transfuse over no more than 4 hours ▲ Typically over 60 minutes
Cryoprecipitate	To replace: ▲ **Fibrinogen:** In patients actively bleeding who have a low fibrinogen level	Frozen **1 year** Once thawed expires after 4 hours stored at 20-24° C	▲ Blood tubing required ▲ Transfuse as rapidly as tolerated

Appendix 2: Blood products table (list not comprehensive)

Blood Product	Major Uses	Storage & Expiration	Administration
Albumin (5% and 25%)	25%: ▲ Ascites patients undergoing large volume paracentesis greater than 5 litres ▲ Spontaneous Bacterial Peritonitis (SBP) ▲ Hepatorenal syndrome 5%: ▲ Plasma exchange procedures	Room temperature < 30° C Expires as indicated on packaging	▲ Standard IV set with vent ▲ No blood tubing or filtering required ▲ Begin infusion slowly then as tolerated ▲ Maximum rate: • Albumin 25% - 120 mL/hr • Albumin 5% - 300 mL/hr (excluding exchange procedures)
Intravenous Immune Globulin (IVIG)	▲ Replacement of Immunoglobulins ▲ Control of some infections and autoimmune diseases	Storage variable by brand Expires as indicated on packaging	▲ Standard IV set with vent ▲ No blood tubing or filtering required ▲ Infusion pump required ▲ Begin infusion slowly and increase as tolerated ▲ For maximum rate – check package insert/hospital policy as brand specific ▲ Frequent vital sign monitoring required

Blood Product	Major Uses	Storage & Expiration	Administration
Rh Immune Globulin (RhIG)	Used for Rh negative patients: ▲ Following exposure or possible exposure to Rh positive blood ▲ To prevent sensitization to the Rh(D) antigen during pregnancy	2-8° C Expires as indicated on packaging	▲ Administered usually IM but may be given IV
	▲ Treatment of non-splenectomized Rh positive patients with Immune Thrombocytopenic Purpura (ITP)		▲ Administered IV through a standard IV set ▲ May be given slow push usually by physician
Prothrombin Complex Concentrate (PCC)	▲ Urgent reversal of warfarin (Coumadin®) or Vitamin K deficiency in bleeding patients and those requiring emergency surgery	2-25° C Expires as indicated on packaging Use immediately once reconstituted	▲ Standard IV set with vent ▲ No blood tubing or filtering required ▲ Usually infused over 15 - 30 minutes (brand specific) ▲ May be given slow push usually by physician ▲ Dosage based on patient weight and INR value, usually 2 - 4 vials (500 IU per vial) ▲ Effect is immediate and lasts 6 - 12 hours ▲ For complete reversal, Vitamin K 10 mg IV must also be given

Appendix 3: Compatibility chart

PATIENT BLOOD GROUP	COMPATIBLE DONOR BLOOD GROUP			
	Red Blood Cells	Platelets	Plasma/ Cryosupernatant Plasma**	Cryoprecipitate**
O Positive	O Positive O Negative	Rh Positive or Negative O preferred	Any Group	Any Group
O Negative*	O Negative	Rh Negative O preferred	Any Group	Any Group
A Positive	A Positive, A Negative O Positive, O Negative	Rh Positive or Negative A preferred	A, AB	Any Group
A Negative*	A Negative O Negative	Rh Negative A preferred	A, AB	Any Group
B Positive	B Positive, B Negative O Positive, O Negative	Rh Positive or Negative B preferred	B, AB	Any Group
B Negative*	B Negative O Negative	Rh Negative B preferred	B, AB	Any Group
AB Positive	Any Group Positive/Negative	Rh Positive or Negative AB preferred	AB	Any Group
AB Negative*	Any Group Negative	Rh Negative AB preferred	AB	Any Group

* In urgent situations (or during times of shortages) Rh Negative patients may need to receive Rh Positive RBCs and Platelets

** Rh of plasma and cryoprecipitate is not relevant and no longer appears on CBS label

Universal RBC for urgent transfusion:
▲ O Negative for females less than 45 years
▲ O Positive for all others

Universal Plasma for urgent transfusion:
▲ AB

Appendix 4: Canadian Blood Services label

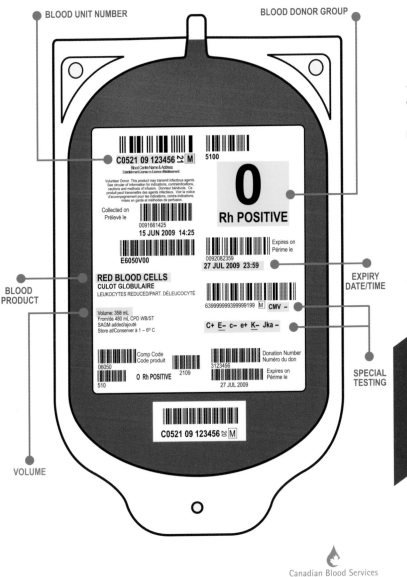

BLOOD UNIT NUMBER

BLOOD DONOR GROUP

C0521 09 123456 21 M

5100

Blood Centre Name & Address
Établissment/Licence n°/Licence/Établissement

Volunteer Donor. This product may transmit infectious agents.
See circular of information for indications, contraindications,
cautions and methods of infusion. Donneur bénévole. Ce
produit peut transmettre des agents infectieux. Voir la notice
d'accompagnement pour les indications, contre-indications,
mises en garde et méthodes de perfusion.

Collected on
Prélevé le

0091661425
15 JUN 2009 14:25

E6050V00

RED BLOOD CELLS
CULOT GLOBULAIRE
LEUKOCYTES REDUCED/PART. DÉLEUCOCYTÉ

Volume: 358 mL
From/de 480 mL CPD WB/ST
SAGM added/ajouté
Store at/Conserver à 1 – 6° C

BLOOD
PRODUCT

Comp Code
Code produit
06050

O Rh POSITIVE   2109

510

VOLUME

0

Rh POSITIVE

Expires on
Périme le
0092082359
27 JUL 2009 23:59

EXPIRY
DATE/TIME

639999999399999199   M   CMV –

C+ E– c– e+ K– Jka –

SPECIAL
TESTING

Donation Number
Numéro du don
3123456

Expires on
Périme le
27 JUL 2009

C0521 09 123456 20 M

43

Appendix 5: Acute reactions - risk and description table

ACUTE TRANSFUSION REACTION	RISK OF EVENT
Minor allergic reaction	1 in 100
Anaphylaxis	1 in 40,000
Febrile Non-Hemolytic (transfusion reaction per unit of RBC)	1 in 300
Bacterial Sepsis (per platelet concentrate)	1 in 10,000 will become symptomatic 1 in 60,000 will be fatal
Bacterial Sepsis (per unit of RBC)	1 in 250,000 will become symptomatic 1 in 500,000 will be fatal
Acute Hemolytic Transfusion Reaction	1 in 40,000
Transfusion Related Acute Lung Injury (TRALI)	1 in 12,000
Transfusion Associated Circulatory Overload (TACO)	1 in 100
Hypotensive Reaction	Very Rare

DESCRIPTION

Mild allergic reaction to an allergen in the blood component/product.

Potentially fatal reaction caused by an allergen that the patient has been sensitized to.

Mild usually self-limiting reaction associated with donor white blood cells or cytokines in the blood component/product. Usually presents with fever and/or rigors (shaking).

Potentially fatal reaction caused by bacteria inadvertently introduced into the blood component/product or originating from the donor. More common in platelets due to room temperature storage.

Potentially fatal reaction caused by blood group incompatibility. Results in hemolysis of the incompatible transfused RBCs or of the patient's own RBCs if incompatible plasma and rarely platelets are transfused. Can also be caused by chemical hemolysis (e.g., mixing with incompatible medications or solutions) or mechanical hemolysis (e.g., cell savers, transfusing rapidly through a too small needle, improper storage). Can result in renal failure, shock and coagulopathy.

Acute hypoxemia with evidence of new bilateral lung infiltrates on X-Ray and no evidence of circulatory overload. Patients often require ventilatory support. Etiology not fully understood. Postulated to be caused by donor antibodies (anti-HLA or anti-HNA)* interacting with recipient antigens or vice versa. Usually occurs within 1-2 hours of start of transfusion and rarely after 6 hours. Usually resolves within 24-72 hours with death occurring in 5-10% of cases.

Circulatory overload from excessively rapid transfusion and/or in patients at greater risk for overload (e.g., very young, elderly, impaired cardiac function). Preventative measures include slower transfusion rates and pre-emptive diuretics for patients at risk.

Bradykinin mediated hypotension. Characterized by profound drop in blood pressure usually seen in patients on ACE Inhibitors unable to degrade bradykinin in blood component/product.

*Anti-HLA and anti-HNA antibodies can develop after exposure to blood or through pregnancies
HLA – Human Leukocyte Antigen – antigens located on white blood cells and platelets
HNA – Human Neutrophil Antigen – antigens located on neutrophils

SIGNS AND SYMPTOMS		USUAL TIMING	POSSIBLE ETIOLOGY
Fever (at least 38° C and an increase of at least 1° C from baseline) **and/or** Shaking Chills/Rigors	38°C to 38.9°C but **NO** other symptoms	During or up to 4 hours post transfusion	Febrile non-hemolytic transfusion reaction
	Less than 39°C but with other symptoms (e.g., rigors, hypotension) **or** 39° C or more	Usually within first 15 minutes but may be later	Febrile non-hemolytic transfusion reaction Bacterial contamination Acu te hemolytic transfusion reaction
Urticaria (hives)	Less than 2/3 body but **NO** other symptoms	During or up to 4 hours post transfusion	Minor allergic
Itching **or** Rash	2/3 body or more but **NO** other symptoms	Usually early in transfusion	Minor allergic (extensive)
	Accompanied by other symptoms (e.g., dyspnea hypotension)	Usually early in transfusion	Anaphylactoid reaction/Anaphylaxis
Dyspnea **or** Decrease in SpO$_2$% to 90% or less (and a change of at least 5% from baseline)	Typically with hypertension	Within several hours of transfusion	Transfusion associated circulatory overload (TACO)
	Typically with hypotension	Within 6 hours of transfusion	Transfusion related acute lung injury (TRALI)
		Usually within first 15 minutes but may be later	Bacterial contamination Acute hemolytic transfusion reaction Anaphylaxis

Appendix 6: Transfusion reaction chart

TTISS ON

Developed by Ontario Transfusion Transmitted Injuries Surveillance System (TTISS-ON)
Version 2 November 2015

Recommended Investigations	Suggested Treatment and Actions
No testing required	▲ Antipyretic ▲ With physician approval transfusion may be resumed cautiously if product still viable
▲ Group & Screen, DAT ▲ Patient blood culture(s) ▲ Urinalysis If hemolysis suspected (e.g., red urine or plasma) ▲ CBC, electrolytes, creatinine, bilirubin, LDH aPTT, INR, fibrinogen, haptoglobin, plasma Hb	**Do not restart transfusion** ▲ Antipyretic ▲ Consider Meperidine (Demerol®) for significant rigors ▲ If bacterial contamination suspected, antibiotics should be started immediately ▲ Monitor for hypotension, renal failure and DIC ▲ Return blood product to Transfusion Laboratory ▲ For additional assistance, contact _____
No testing required	▲ Antihistamine ▲ With physician approval transfusion may be resumed cautiously if product still viable
No testing required	**Do not restart transfusion** ▲ Antihistamine ▲ May require steroid
▲ Group & Screen, DAT ▲ Chest X-Ray (if dyspneic) ▲ Blood gases (if dyspneic) ▲ Haptoglobin ▲ Anti-IgA testing	**Do not restart transfusion** ▲ Epinephrine ▲ Washed/plasma depleted blood products pending investigation ▲ Return blood product to Transfusion Laboratory ▲ For additional assistance, contact _____
▲ Group & Screen, DAT ▲ Chest X-Ray ▲ Blood gases ▲ Urinalysis	**Do not restart transfusion** ▲ Diuretics, oxygen, High Fowler's position ▲ Return blood product to Transfusion Laboratory ▲ Slow transfusion rate with diuretics for future transfusions
If sepsis suspected: ▲ Patient blood culture(s) If hemolysis suspected: ▲ CBC, electrolytes, creatinine, bilirubin, LDH aPTT, INR, fibrinogen, haptoglobin, plasma Hb If anaphylaxis suspected: ▲ Haptoglobin, Anti-IgA	**Do not restart transfusion** ▲ Assess chest X-Ray for bilateral pulmonary infiltrates ▲ If TRALI may require vasopressors and respiratory support ▲ If bacterial contamination suspected, antibiotics should be started immediately ▲ Monitor for hypotension, renal failure and DIC ▲ If anaphylaxis suspected, epinephrine ▲ Return blood product to Transfusion Laboratory ▲ For additional assistance, contact _____